10 Proven Secrets To Permanent Weight Loss

You Can Be Happy And Feel Great While Losing Weight.

It's Easier Than You Think!

ELLE GARNER

www.MyTakePress.com
www.ElleGarner.com

Published by: **My Take Press**
http://MyTakePress.com

TABLE OF CONTENTS

INTRODUCTION

This book will likely be controversial.

I want you to know up front that I am not a medical professional, nutritionist, or a personal trainer. I don't have specialized qualifications to write this book, and what you're about to read is *my personal story*, and the **10 Proven Secrets** that finally made the difference in my permanent weight loss journey.

My story in a nutshell is that I was forty pounds overweight. I lost that weight – and I kept it off. Not for a few weeks, or a few months, or even a year -- but for more than *twenty* years.

Up until that point I read many, many diet books, and tried so many different diets and fads that I lost count. Literally.

I tried everything except maybe the most bizarre things (ok, well maybe I tried a few of those, too) to lose weight. The sad reality is that none of them worked for any length of time. Oh, I lost weight with some of them – but I always gained it back.

Then one day I decided to stop spinning my wheels on the perpetual vicious cycle of fad diets once and for all.

I didn't have an advantage over you...

- I'm not an athlete.
- I couldn't afford a personal trainer.
- I don't have "good genes".
- I didn't have a personal chef.
- I don't have incredible will power.

I struggled much of my life with being over weight to some degree or another.

Then I *determined* it was **not** going to be that way for the rest of my life. I read, and I researched, and I read some more. I began the journey by adopting a healthy plan for eating where the food I ate would largely nourish my body.

But that still isn't what made the difference.

It took time, but I found what I believe are THE secrets to true weight loss for LIFE.

I created a plan that worked – a plan that fostered a new relationship with my body, food, and eating patterns. It worked so well that I kept the weight off *permanently*.

What's the downside?

- It's simple – but not easy.
- It is not a magic pill, and I don't have a magic wand that will help you lose weight.
- I can't lose the weight for you.
- Reading this book won't make you lose weight either. (It will not happen by osmosis.)

Like me, you will have to make some decisions along the way that will determine if this is right for you, and if you're willing to do it -- **Every. Single. Day.**

What I can promise you is that if you do exactly what I did - what I share with you in this book - you will realize a healthy weight for your body.

Does that sound bold? It is. I'm confident because I'm living, breathing, happy, and healthy proof.

Are there exceptions? Sure.

Some people have medical complications and issues that impact their body's ability to reach a healthy weight. If that's your situation, I believe this book will still help you have a more healthy relationship with your body, and with food - but I will not promise you that you will lose weight.

AND: *If you haven't consulted with your doctor or health care provider regarding an exercise and weight loss program, please do so BEFORE you start this or any program.*

Here's some good news: you will not need to spend one dime beyond the cost of this book to learn or put the **10 Proven Secrets** into practice.

That's right. I'm giving you *everything* right here.

I'm not going to give you one piece of what I did, and then ask you buy the rest of the details in book 2, or book 3, or book 4 and beyond. You're getting it all. Does that mean I will never write another book on this topic? No. I'm passionate about this *and* empowering others to do whatever it takes to get healthy.

But you won't need to purchase anything else from me in order to get ALL **10 Proven Secrets**. This book contains exactly what you need to do in order to follow what worked for me.

The weight loss industry is a <u>multi-billion dollar business</u>; it makes sense that some people want you to believe that the process of losing weight *has to be hard.*

They want you to believe that the secret to weight loss is their DVD or expensive exercise equipment.

It's not.

More fallacies – or 'YoYo Plans' as I call them:

- We need diet plans that require monthly fees and prepackaged meals. (That fosters dependence and leads you to believe that you can't make your own food choices and lose weight. Simply not true.)
- You need to sweat hard, eat little, and be really miserable in order to lose weight. (How many of us will actually do that? Not me.)
- You need special shakes, pills, or a plan that forces you count every calorie and point in order to lose weight. (Not so.)

I tried all of those – and none of them worked for me long term.

Like many people, there was always something standing in my way. It wasn't for lack of trying or motivation! It wasn't the foods I was eating or the exercises I had chosen.

So what was it?

Over time, I was able to uncover that what worked for me was actually transforming the way that I think about food and weight loss as a whole, and creating new patterns, paradigms and beliefs around food and the purpose of food in my life.

Adjusting my mindset was critical. This meant that I had to *transform* how I looked at food, hunger, my weight, health, adequate water and exercise.

In this book, we're going to talk about what I learned during the process of shedding those extra pounds and staying at an optimal weight long-term. This isn't about a crash diet or some fad that will only be popular for a few weeks or months. Instead, this is about a transformation from the inside out state that will make weight loss easier, it will change how you look at hunger and food, and help you keep it off permanently and naturally - yes with just **10 Proven Secrets**.

As you tap into this, and you begin to have power over what you eat and when you eat, you will be amazed at the personal freedom and joy that begins to take the place of food and weight struggles.

Sound good? It is! **Let's get started.**

THE TRUTH ABOUT WEIGHT LOSS

The truth about weight loss is that your obesity or overweight state is largely a physical manifestation of bad habits, beliefs, mindset, and mind*less*ness.

Think that's an oversimplification? Read on.

For someone to actually lose weight and keep it off long-term - mindset must change, how we listen to our body must change, and our patterns must change. Once you do this, many other things in your life will change along with it.

If you really want permanent weight loss, you have to make this shift or risk regaining back all the weight. I'm sure you've heard that it takes high amounts of willpower to lose weight and keep it off. Honestly, I *disagree*.

Trying to white knuckle your way to success when it comes to long-term weight loss doesn't work. It isn't fun. It doesn't truly change anything, and that approach doesn't result in permanent weight loss.

Sure, you could knock 10, 20 or maybe even 100 pounds off of your frame, but will you keep it off long-term with just willpower?

The chances are that you won't because really, who WANTS to live like THAT? Eventually almost everyone falls back into old patterns and emotional eating habits in the long run.

Though willpower is a strong part of how your brain works, you also have natural inclinations in your body that will overcome willpower at every turn.

Great, so what *does* work?

Transforming your mindset, patterns, and relationship with your body and food. Sound simple? It is - and it isn't.

A new mindset also means new ways of looking at yourself, food, exercise/movement - and this often results in a change in the *way* that you do things.

- You learn how to properly plan your meals and move your body.
- You learn how to overcome emotional moments with something other than food.
- You learn replacements for bad habits instead of trying the white knuckle, willpower-fueled method of avoiding something, or worse yet, unhealthy weight loss methods and pills.
- You learn to appreciate food, and what it can do **for** your body.
- You learn to *love* how your body feels as you *listen.*
- YOU will be empowered.
- This is life-changing stuff – at least it was for me.

As you can scc from just these few examples, weight loss is more about your mindset, psychological growth, and getting in touch with your body, than it is about how much weight you lift and what you eat for lunch today or tomorrow.

When you learn **how to use your mind to transform your core beliefs around food, hunger and moving your body** -- you are unstoppable!

Never again will food and excessive eating have a hold on you because your relationship with yourself, food and exercise will change inside of you, in a way that feels so right and good.

It's my experience and opinion that you won't ever want to return to the way you were before.

TRANSFORMING YOUR MIND

When you hear someone say that you have to reprogram or transform your mind to successfully lose weight, you might feel like it's a bit "out there". I can assure this isn't some new age thing we're talking about here. We're talking about something that is real, tangible and within your reach.

We're talking about using the subconscious power of the human mind to transform and renew how you think and feel about your body, food, patterns, and exercise. Your subconscious mind is far more powerful that you realize – trust me on this! The mind is an incredibly powerful force in your life, and much more powerful than the next diet plan or workout DVD.

From a nutritional perspective, the book that began my journey of influence and transformation was Dr. Andrew Weil's book called "Eating Well For Optimal Health". It challenged my thinking and gave clear guidelines on healthy food, nutrition, and how your body gets energy from food. I highly recommend it.

However, just reading a book about nutrition wasn't going to get me to my end goal. Instead, I also had to do some research on completely adjusting my mindset, and even subconscious mind, so that I could learn how to eat mindfully and get in touch with my body.

I had to explore my own relationship with food and why I made the choices I did with food, inactivity, my health, and nutrition choices (or lack thereof).

One of the best ways to transform your mind and belief system around healthy weight, weight loss, and food is by acknowledging the truth about your beliefs relative to hunger, food and nutrition – by daily practicing the following **10 Proven Secrets *DAILY*** – *exactly* as is outlined here.

These 10 Proven Secrets enforce both the behavior you want to change and the results you desire COMBINED with choices to honor these affirmatively.

After extensive research, I came up with my list of **10 Secrets**.

I read them meditatively on a *daily basis* when my subconscious mind was most open to influence - **when I first woke up, immediately before going to sleep at night, and whenever I needed to throughout the day**.

I wrote these transformational secrets on 5 x 8 index cards, and put one on my nightstand, in the kitchen, on the fridge, in my office, and even in my handbag. I made sure that *wherever* I was I could read the 10 Secrets and reinforce these new beliefs and behaviors.

Let's take a look a closer look.

THE 10 PROVEN SECRETS

This is KEY!! Write these 10 Secrets down on a 5 x 8 index card, or type them up. (When you get to the end of this book, you'll find a free bonus that will help you with this step!)

NOW Read them when you...

1. FIRST wake in the morning
2. Throughout the day as needed
3. Again right before falling asleep at night

Do This Every Single Day.

This is *essential* for success. Commit to doing this every day, and you will begin to see changes; changes in your awareness of your body, in your attitude toward eating, in your attitude toward food, and yes, even in your waistline and weight *loss*.

Ready? Here they are!

1. I eat only when my body is hungry.

You've heard this before, but it is very helpful for you to <u>write these down right now</u>.

Follow the instructions above and read this *minimally* when you **first wake** and **right before falling asleep at night**, and then as needed **throughout the day**.

If you start to feel like you need to eat, but you know it's either from boredom, stress, or emotion and not true physical hunger, read these secrets. Get in touch with your body and when you are truly hungry.

How do you do this? Well, start by committing TODAY (and each day thereafter) that you will only eat when you actually feel very hungry. It's easy to confuse thirst or an emotional response with hunger.

Get to know your body. Reacquaint yourself with what your stomach and body feels like when it's actually HUNGRY.

Some people are so afraid of hunger that they never even allow themselves to feel hunger, or what hungry is really like.

Take inventory. Are you actually hungry? Remind yourself that you should only be eating food when your body is really and truly hungry.

While this might seem like a very basic thing, it's important to realize that many of us eat for many reasons that have nothing to do with hunger.

We eat because it is "time to eat" or because everyone else is eating, but we may not actually be physically hungry.

Eating only when you are hungry is a BIG step toward being successful with weight loss, a healthy body weight, and a healthy relationship with food.

Start this step right now. Wait until you're *really* hungry to eat.

2. I eat in a calm environment. Reduce distractions.

This is one of those rules that is most easily broken, especially in light of the busy lives most of us lead today.

We eat in front of the television set, or while we're on the run, in the midst of chaos, or even during our commute to or from work. Instead, sit down at the table to really enjoy every meal you eat with intention and mindfulness.

Many people sit down in front of the TV with a bag of chips, and before they know it their hand hits the bottom of the bag. That's one example of mind*less* eating – and it's responsible for a lot of extra and empty calories that we don't need.

Studies have proven that when we eat in a calm environment, our body assimilates the foods and nutrients AND we gain the benefit of consciously realizing that we are eating.

Savor your food – enjoy it.

3. I eat only when I'm sitting.

Many of us are in the habit of eating while were standing, or on the run, or we simply graze on food throughout the day. If this is you – stop!

Make your meals an event. Are you about to eat? Are you sitting? If not, SIT.

Sit down at the table and actually enjoy your food instead of rushing or multi-tasking while you eat.

Even when you eat snacks, make sure that you treat them with respect just like a meal. Create your snack-sized portions in advance so that they are always there to grab quickly, but eat them sitting down and follow all of these 10 Secret Steps any time you eat – whether it's a meal or snack.

If you're going to eat anything no matter how large or how small – SIT.

4. I eat only if my body and mind are relaxed.

It might be difficult to imagine a time where you're stress-free, but this is the state your mind and body should be in before you eat.

Only eat when you're relaxed. If you're about to eat and you're not relaxed, take a moment to breath. Practice this:

When you breath in, think about breathing in relaxation and when you breathe out, think about breathing out and releasing your stress. Do this a few times prior to eating and I guarantee – you will notice a difference, and you will be more relaxed.

If we eat when stressed, we risk eating out of emotion instead of true physical hunger AND our body simply cannot process the food as well.

So, don't eat when you are stressed out, angry, sad, mad, etc. Calm yourself through prayer, meditation, breathing or even yoga.

5. I eat and drink only food and beverages my body LOVES.

Wow! Have you ever read this in any "diet plan"?

We're conditioned that when we go on a diet, we have to eat food that we hate. Often we dread the thought of our next meal because we know it's not even going to be food we like.

Does this sound like a successful weight loss program to you?

When I decided to take control of my life and lose the excess weight my body didn't need or want - I only ate food that my body loved.

Honestly.

How did I do this? Well, the foods you eat will be different from the foods I ate, but if you follow all the steps and 10 Secrets that I am outlining here, you will absolutely notice your relationship with food, and your body begin to change.

I found that I didn't eat nearly as much or even crave the unhealthy foods I had before – because I ate them if I wanted to. But I only ate them if I was hungry, and calm, and sitting, and following the rest of the secrets you're about to read below.

I'm telling you – this works – and it's liberating!

Eating what you love naturally makes you enjoy the food you eat, and you feel satisfied when you eat. No more deprivation.

6. I pay attention only to my food when eating.

Okay, if you are a parent you are probably thinking about putting this book down right about now. How is it even possible to pay attention only to your food when you have small children sitting at the table with you?

You've probably noticed by now that all of these secrets are following a similar path. It's about slowing down and really focusing on the food you're eating rather than external events, people, or devices.

If you have children, do you think they will benefit from learning these secrets early in their life? You bet they will! In fact, if you teach them this as you are learning it, they will likely avoid the challenges you are facing right now.

Children LOVE secrets – most of us do. If you have children, here's one approach I recommend.

- Sit down with your kids and talk about this book.
- Make it FUN and serious. Be excited.
- Tell them you've found 10 Secrets that are going to help you have a healthy body and weight – are they game to know these secrets too?
- ASK if they'll help with your secret pact.
- Prepare yourself for the fact that this will be a challenge – and be prepared for it. How? Have the 10 Secrets on your table, and when someone "forgets" one of them, very quietly remind them that Secret #6 (or whichever one it is) is out! Oops.
- Be kind with them and yourself.

Have you ever eaten an entire meal while watching something particularly interesting on TV – only to find that you don't even remember tasting or eating most of your food? Have you ever driven to work or another destination and realized you covered a portion of the drive without even being aware that you had?

When you pay attention **only to your food** while eating, your mind, body, and subconscious are all consciously aware that you are eating; that you are satisfying your hunger, and providing the food, energy and nutrients that your body needs to survive and function optimally.

7. I eat slowly, savoring each and every bite.

When you slow down and actually taste the food you're eating, you'll be aware that your hunger has been satisfied faster.

In fact, the body has a mechanism that releases a specific hormone to let you know when you're full – or nearly full. This usually happens about 20 minutes into a meal.

When we eat slowly, chew our food well, and savor the food we're eating, it gives our body and mind the chance to catch up with the fact that we are fulfilling that need and hunger signal.

I know this sounds basic, but if you really think about it you'll see the logic behind it.

It is possible to go through a day, and each and every day, without ever eating mindfully. Many of us do it constantly. When we do this, we never consciously acknowledge that we've eaten or met our body's need for food and nutrition, because we're eating while thinking about something else or doing something else.

THIS step is so important, in combination with all the other steps. Eat your food slowly so that your body has time to recognize that you are meeting this need and honoring your hunger.

If this is hard for you, make the conscious choice to chew each bite of food at least 20 times before you swallow. Why? For one thing, it slows you down and gives your mind and body the chance to sync. Secondly, when you chew your food thoroughly, your mouth releases enzymes that help your digestive system break the food down. Proper digestion is critical for health and weight loss.

You will be amazed at the tastes you rediscover, and the flavors that you missed before while mindlessly swallowing whatever was in your mouth.

8. I stop eating before my body is full.

If you eat too fast, you miss the signals your body gives you when it's satisfied. When we eat slowly and consciously, we give ourselves the chance to tune into our body, and learn to read when we've had enough. This is a critical step to stopping *well before* you get to that stuffed feeling.

Some people have no idea what "before full" or "satisfied" means until they are stuffed and uncomfortable. They eat and eat, and then they are miserable when they are stuffed and can't keep their pants buttoned or zipped.

Listen and learn your body's cues. Figure out when "satisfied" happens for you. If you are eating slowly, it will be a lot easier to recognize.

Be curious about this, and aware. As yourself, "What is the point where my body is satisfied?"

9. I drink a full glass of water before eating.

This is SO important! Many of us are dehydrated and simply do not drink enough *pure* WATER. If you drink a full glass of pure water (at least 8 ounces) before eating, it will do two things.

One, it will help you determine if you are actually hungry or simply thirsty. Many of us confuse this, and eat when we're actually thirsty. It's important to learn the difference and drinking a full glass of water before eating any meal will help you achieve this.

Two, it will give your body a sense of fullness and you will eat less than you might otherwise – if you are truly listening to the signals from your body.

Tune in.

Our body needs a certain amount of water each day in order to function properly and detoxify. Doing this every day before you put any food in your mouth will help you begin to understand the difference between thirst and hunger. It's confused far more often that you might think.

10. I move my body for 15 to 30 minutes daily, 5 days per week.

MOVE!

Studies are substantiating that people who move throughout the day are stronger, happier, and have fewer health challenges.

I'm NOT an advocate for aerobics or hard-core exercise – unless that is something you truly enjoy.

Honestly, if you don't truly enjoy it you will not stick with it.

We have to be physically active in order to create and support a healthy body.

Find activities that you love to do. Don't do exercises that you hate because that sends the wrong message to your mind and body, and it's not likely to last long.

Take chances and try new things because you may actually like something and you won't know until you try it.

Start slowly if you have been sedentary for a long time, and *please* **check with your doctor before starting any new exercise or weight loss program**.

*   *   *

You can stop right here, commit to following these steps and be successful at attaining a weight that is healthy for your body!

In combination, these steps will change your eating patterns, and the way you perceive hunger and food. Even if you only read these **10 Proven Secrets** first thing in the morning upon waking, and again right before falling asleep at night – it will make a difference.

If you read them additionally throughout the day as needed, it will take your success with this system up a notch.

Please believe me and try it – because it WORKS!! It really does.

If you want a deeper understanding of the principles behind these ten steps and how they work, read on. I think you'll find the information here helpful in establishing a basis for why this works.

If not, and if you are ready to get started, go to the last chapter in this book to learn how to access the free bonus I'm providing – a beautiful list of the 10 Secrets that you can print and take with you wherever you go. Put it on your nightstand, in your bathroom, on your fridge, in your handbag or briefcase, in your office, etc.

I make it easy for you to print multiple copies of this list and have it accessible whenever you need it – and minimally at the times specified.

MINDFUL EATING

As you can see, many of the Secrets listed above are largely about mindful eating. Mindful eating simply means that you actually think about what you're eating and focus on the food while you have it in front of you.

There's no question that we are a scattered society. Everyone is overstressed and overscheduled. While it's very tempting to run through the drive-through or eat in your car on the way home from work, it's not the best thing for your overall health. How can you properly focus on your food when you are distracted by other things? When you don't concentrate, you eat past your 'satisfied limits' and continue the bad habit of not paying attention to your body's signals.

Mindful eating means that you make time to have actual meals and you sit down to focus on the food in front of you. You chew slowly and enjoy each bite. You don't get distracted or stressed out during a meal. Eating becomes a spiritual experience rather than something that you do without even thinking about it.

When was the last time you actually enjoyed the meal you were eating? Think about that for a moment. When did you really taste the food and appreciate the fact that you were eating it? I'm not talking about a fast food hamburger. I am talking about a meal that had flavor and smells and richness that made you literally close your eyes and savor it.

USING FOOD AS FUEL

When you make the shift to understanding that your body needs to use food as fuel, you better appreciate what you're putting in it. Just like you wouldn't run your car using liquefied lard, you shouldn't put that in your body either.

Our bodies are machines, and we want them to work for many years to come. I don't know anyone who wants to live a short life, do you? If you want to live a long and healthy life, it's important to learn how to use food as fuel instead of an emotional crutch. You need a variety of nutrients and building blocks in your body such as carbohydrates, proteins and fats. Yes, I said carbs! Many people try to avoid a particular component, but our bodies need them. The problem comes in when you focus too much on one thing to the exclusion of other things. We're talking about balance here. (And of course, I recommend whole grain carbs, when you choose to eat them.)

We all have certain triggers that cause us to want to overeat. Most of these are rooted in family, genetics and to some degree even the media. Everyone needs to explore this personally in order to find the root of his or her personal beliefs as it relates to food.

For me, I ate emotionally. For some reason I also had a very primitive attitude toward food, and I acted like I should eat as much as I could in the moment, as if there wouldn't be enough for tomorrow or the next meal.

The crazy thing is that I had never gone hungry. I'm not sure where that belief came from, but it plagued me for years.

Another belief that I had about food was that I needed to eat everything on my plate. That one definitely came from my mom! A lot of people have the belief that they must "be a member of the clean plate club". Some mothers and fathers even use guilt as a way of getting kids to eat everything on their plates by saying that children in other parts of the world aren't so lucky to have food. However, this just sets kids up for disaster when it comes to eating because it tells them to eat whether they are hungry or even like the food on their plates.

The most freeing principal that I eventually realized was that I could eat anything I wanted. Really! I could eat anything I wanted and it was okay, especially if I applied the 10 Secrets Steps to my eating. Nothing was off limits.

No matter what your trigger(s) are, you have to learn how to recognize them and then use it as a way of turning this weight-loss shipwreck around. If you continue to honor erroneous beliefs, you'll let them rule your life as you continue to struggle with weight loss.

Trust me, you don't need them. Let them go.

EMOTIONAL EATING

Let's take a quick moment to talk a little bit about emotional eating since it is a problem that many of us have, regardless of whether we are male or female.

In fact, I would venture to guess that most of the over weight people in the world are emotional eaters, whether they realize it or not. It's one thing to like food, but it's quite another to gorge on it when you know it is harmful to your health.

In its simplest form, emotional eating means that you're eating for reasons other than hunger. Instead of being physically hungry, you are using emotional triggers to propel you to eat.

So how do you tell the difference between emotional hunger and physical hunger?

The first thing to remember is that emotional hunger comes on suddenly while physical hunger occurs gradually as your stomach empties. When you are physically hungry, you will have signs and symptoms as you become hungrier. You may even get shaky from low blood sugar (although it is NEVER wise to let your body get to this point!). This is a gradual thing unlike emotional eating which can make you feel like you have to eat right now or you will lose it.

Also, when you're eating emotionally, you'll typically crave a specific food or type of food. For instance, you might crave ice cream or a hamburger. When you're physically hungry, you'll eat just about anything because you're trying to fill a biological need. When it's emotional eating, you look at many different options instead of eating what is available.

Emotional hunger feels like you must satisfy it instantly with a specific food that you crave. Physical hunger can actually wait until food is available.

Let's look at an example of this. Let's say that you just had a particularly rough day at work and you start craving pizza. If you are physically hungry, you go to your refrigerator and find whatever food is available and make that work. If you're really emotionally hungry, you get the phone book and immediately call the local pizza parlor to have your food delivered.

Emotional eating is an immature way of looking at life and food. You want to immediately satisfy your cravings like a kid having a temper tantrum at the toy store.

When you're emotionally hungry, you'll often eat until you feel stuffed. In other words, you're not eating to satisfy a physical hunger. You often won't stop when you're full. Think of a wild animal; do you see them gorging all day long without stopping? You never see a monkey eating banana after banana until he feels like he is going to pop. That's because animals aren't eating out of emotion. They are eating out of physical hunger, so they stop when they are satisfied.

Finally, emotional eating will often make you feel guilty while physical hunger doesn't. (Was that an "ah ha" moment for you?) When you eat out of physical hunger, you're simply giving your body the fuel that it needs to function. Emotional eating may cause you to hide food and feel guilty later.

CHECK IN WITH YOURSELF

Here are some of the questions I ask myself before I eat so that I can check in with myself to make sure that I'm eating out of **real physical hunger** and not emotional cravings. (This is something you will find you only need to do initially because as you follow the steps in this book, you'll soon develop a deeper understanding and ability to read and honor your body's signals.)

First, I ask myself **if I'm hungry**. If the answer is no, than I'll have a glass of water and wait to eat until I am.

Be honest with yourself here because emotional hunger is the one driving factors that I believe makes most people overweight in the first place. **It's not physical hunger that's making you fat**. Your body knows when it's really hungry and when it's not, so reprogramming your mind to know when emotional eating is at the steering wheel is critical.

Next, I ask **if I am in a calm environment**. If not, I will wait until I am in a calm environment before I eat. If I'm really hungry, I'll go to a place where I can be in a calm environment. Calm doesn't mean you need to eat in a meditation room. It just means don't eat in a room full of chaos where your emotional eating tendencies could overwhelm you.

Then I'll check in - **am I sitting**? If not, I'll hold off until I can sit and relax while I'm eating. Don't walk around while you're eating – or stand. Even at buffets or work functions, find a chair and sit in it. Be calm, relaxed, and mindful when eating.

If you can't be – then just enjoy being social! Maybe eat before you leave for an event, just enough so you are not hungry, and then enjoy the chance to really connect with people at your event. You might be surprised at how freeing it is, and how much more observant you are.

Another important question to ask is, **do you *love* what you're about to eat**? Or are you just eating to eat?

If you're going to eat, you might as well love it! Personally, if I don't love what I am about to eat, I will forgo it for the time being until I can get what I actually want to eat.

Is my mind and body relaxed - or am I feeling stressed? If I'm stressed, I use breathing or prayer to calm my spirit and then examine if I'm actually hungry. If I'm hungry, I find something that I love to eat. If I'm not hungry, I move on to do something else.

Another important point is **that I pay attention only to the food I'm eating**. As a side note here, I always try to be thankful for food and ask God's blessing on it. Creating an attitude of gratitude and blessing before I eat allows me to really think about my food and my body. It helps me be aware of what I'm eating and that I'm filling the need that my body has for nourishment and energy. You don't have to be religious or spiritual to adopt this - just take a moment to be grateful before you eat.

Being conscious about this will have enormous impact on your weight loss. Similar to meditation, this one can be tough especially when kids are at the table. Kids will benefit from being aware of their food too, so it's a great thing to practice with the whole family.

My son had a history assignment that required us to create a meal similar to what monks would have eaten before electricity existed. In this instance, the monks were not allowed to talk at all during any meal and only ate by candlelight, as it was all they had. Every day they ate soup, bread and water, and were only allowed to have butter on their bread if it was a holiday or special occasion. (We pretended it was a holiday!)

It was an eye-opening experience for our entire family. It was the first time we had ever sat through a meal without talking before, and to this day it is something we all remember. Creating this kind of atmosphere can actually be fun for your family!

Finally, **I remind myself to stop eating when my body is satisfied and before it is full**. This was another huge piece of the puzzle for me. Since I now allowed myself to eat the foods I love, unlike virtually any diet out there, I didn't have the same desire or need to eat forbidden foods. NO foods are forbidden!

I learned to eat slowly and mindfully, and I became very aware of my body. I soon learned that my body was comfortable, so I didn't worry about when I would get hungry. When I did feel hungry, I followed the above principles and satisfied that hunger.

I want you to understand that these principles were revolutionary for me. It changed my attitude toward food, how I ate, why I ate and brought an amazing balance to my life, health and weight.

From that point on, I no longer struggled with my weight. I didn't even think about it or desire to weigh myself. The evidence was in my clothing and the sizes that I dropped, in a new energy level, and an incredible emotional freedom around food.

I became very in tune with my body, and the benefits were wide spread both physically and emotionally.

Some people may gasp at the fact that no foods were forbidden, but I found that my desire for rich sweets and unhealthy foods lessened. And when I did want something sweet, I had it. Therefore, I would choose to eat a smaller meal to make room for the dessert that I knew I wanted.

I could look at a dessert and think, "Whatever - it will be there later or tomorrow if I choose to eat it then." Sweets and food in general no longer had power over me, but rather, I made choices in sync with what my body truly wanted and needed.

UNIVERSAL BASICS REVIEW

Of course, there are always some universal basics that are recommended for weight loss.

For instance, you definitely need to **drink enough pure water throughout the day** to help detoxify your body and keep you full. Being even slightly dehydrated will make you feel terrible, tired and lightheaded. This is why it's so important to drink at least half of your body weight in ounces of water each day; minimally six to eight glasses of pure water daily.

Understand that I'm not talking about drinking sugary fruit juices, coffee, tea or colas. If you drink those, they will further dehydrate your body causing you to need even more water. In addition, if you're working out, you need to add water above and beyond the figure quoted above.

Personally, when I know I've had the recommended amount of water for the day, then and only then do I tap into my favorite herbal tea or natural beverage.

The second universal basic that you need to remember is that you should **consult your doctor before any exercise or weight loss program.** Your doctor or healthcare provider knows more about your current health status than just about anyone, so make sure that you get their okay before you move forward with any changes to your diet or exercise program.

SLEEP is vital to maintaining a healthy weight and mindset. Get enough sleep every night, and you'll find it supports your movement toward a healthy weight and life!

Finally, you need to **ensure that your weight loss and weight issues are not medically related**. Again, speaking with your doctor is important because he or she will need to make sure that you don't have any extenuating medical circumstances such as Type 2 diabetes or heart disease.

THE PSYCHOLOGY OF WEIGHT LOSS

As mentioned before, weight loss is a multi-billion dollar a year business. It seems like everyone is getting into the fray these days. You have an unlimited number of workout DVDs, and plenty of exercise equipment that you can invest your hard-earned money in.

On top of that, you can buy any number of supposedly healthy weight loss shakes and prepackaged meals that will be delivered right to your front door. No need to spend your time and energy actually cooking a healthy meal when you can pop a nasty-tasting, dehydrated meal into your microwave so that you can pursue your goals of losing weight and eating miserable food.

Many people don't realize that weight loss doesn't have to be so complicated. By learning how to use your mind rather than your money to lose weight, you can create true and lasting change.

We have a tendency to look outside of ourselves when it comes to solutions for health issues, and sometimes that makes sense.

Getting in touch with your body, listening to it and understanding its signals will only better enable you to take care of yourself, or know when you need to seek additional help.

We are born to be healthy and whole, but we get off track because we buy into this modern world's idea of living. We are fast paced, over-scheduled and frankly, UNDER nourished by the fast and processed foods that we consume. For most of us, there's way too much stress in our lives.

When we use the power of our brain to break out of this mindset, our bodies and lives change for the better. It's always there, inside of us, waiting to burst forth and heal our lives. The problem is that we are probably too busy eating a hamburger while texting, while watching TV, and reading a book to notice that the power is inside of us right now!

Unfortunately, there are many people who go to the extreme end of the spectrum and have weight-loss surgery. Many of these people then gain the weight back because they never changed their mindset or patterns. Instead, they look for the quickest road out of being obese by having a potentially deadly weight-loss surgery.

People who have these surgeries end up with lifelong complications in many cases. They can't even absorb nutrients properly anymore, so they have to make sure to stay on specific supplements for life. In addition, they have to eat small amounts of food or risk being nauseous and feeling terrible. Now, if this is you and you have already had surgery – these **10 Proven Secrets** can still help you!

I am explaining this for one reason - weight loss doesn't have to take you to such an extreme end of the spectrum, but even if it has, there's hope.

You can make these simple yet *powerful* changes in your mind, behavior, and relationship with your body so that you don't have to resort to fad diets, starving yourself or working out for hours every day. You don't have to end up under the knife in a cold operating room trying to solve your obesity problem. Often, the answer is between your own ears and choices.

Let's talk a little bit about the psychology of losing weight and what may be going wrong in the process of shedding those extra pounds.

Recent studies have shown that simply dieting isn't a long-term plan for weight loss. In fact, one study showed that less than 20% of obese patients were able to even lose 5% of their body weight and actually keep it off for five years. Part of this is a biological response of the body because it perceives this weight loss to be a starvation situation. This is one of the reasons why researchers don't recommend that people go on very restrictive diets as they can slow metabolism and cause the body to erroneously believe that food is scarce. In the body thinks that food is scarce, it's going to hold on to every ounce and calorie that it can.

On top of that, dieting can also cause people to have a variety of emotional and psychological effects including binge eating, depression, irritability, anxiety and even an obsession over food. Instead of losing weight and keeping it off, the constant focus on what you CAN'T eat causes you to obsess over it, and you end up craving it even more.

It's no surprise that the most effective types of weight-loss programs involve three different things.

First, a change in diet. You obviously have to make some kind of change either of WHAT you are eating or HOW MUCH you are eating. You cannot simply think great thoughts and eat a bowl of ice cream for breakfast, lunch and dinner expecting to look like a supermodel next week. However, if you follow the **10 Proven Secrets** <u>DAILY</u>, you will see that it is VERY hard not to attain a healthy weight no matter what you eating.

For instance, let's say your favorite food in the whole world is French fries. If you eat them at the table, sitting down and eat them slowly paying careful attention to stop before you are full, you will be much better off than eating them mindlessly while you drive home from work. You won't be OVER indulging anymore. You will be enjoying a treat that was eaten after a full glass of water, right? See how they all work together?

Second, add more movement through exercise you enjoy. This isn't a death sentence! You need to find exercises that motivate and excite you. Hate to walk on the treadmill? Then don't! Walk, go dancing, get dance DVDs, join a class, learn to rock climb, buy a bike, start hiking, jump on a mini-trampoline/rebounder…. the options are really only limited by your imagination.

Just MOVE. Your body needs to move whether you want to lose weight or not. Your muscles need it or they atrophy. Your joins need it or they get stiff. Your heart needs it most of all because it is a muscle and needs to work out. Your blood needs to pump and circulate. You need toxins removed. MOVE!

Third is the psychological intervention by way of changing and reprogramming how you think about weight loss and health in general.

Here's the thing that many people don't understand: your mind and body are interconnected. They are not two separate and distinct things. Everything you *think* has a physiological response in your body. When you think a negative thought, you're sending negative energy into the cells of your body. You can actually think your way into sickness and being overweight.

In other words, if you're constantly focused on the fact that you're overweight and unhealthy, you are only attracting more of that because that is where your mind is focused. What you focus on expands. What you sow is also what you'll reap.

Be focused on the outcome that you want. Be focused on mindful eating and daily practicing the **10 Proven Secrets** outlined in this book so that you are headed in a positive direction. Don't stay stuck in the rut of obesity and excess weight. Use your mind – body connection to your advantage.

Some people actually undergo cognitive therapy for weight loss. Cognitive therapy is a well-known psychological method for getting people to break and replace bad habits. For instance, cognitive therapy may include having written reminders on note cards that you carry with you. This is similar to what we talked about earlier.

Many psychologists also offer therapies that are based around the idea of mindfulness. For instance, some counselors are now using something called Mindfulness Based Stress Reduction, which was developed by John Cabot Zinn and his colleagues at Harvard. This method focuses on creating an innate wisdom about food and appetite. Participants in this program are taught how to specifically tune into their own cues of hunger and satiety in their bodies. They are also encouraged to expose themselves to tempting situations, such as going to an all you can eat buffet.

Much like we have discussed, this method of counseling shows people **how to have pleasure in eating** instead of a restrictive attitude. This helps us avoid emotional eating binges and possible depression or anxiety.

Despite what many weight-loss advertisers would want you to believe, there isn't a magic bullet or solution that fits every person. We are all brought up in different situations and have gone through different circumstances in our lives. Our biology and environment is completely different. No one is identical to anyone else even if they're identical twins.

For this reason, there is no specific weight-loss cure that is going to work for every person. Some people are much more likely to regain weight after they've lost it simply because of something hormonal, physical, and or even emotional.

Some people have bodies that have hormone disruptions. Others have problems with emotional eating. Others have depression or anxiety. Maybe you grew up in poverty and didn't have access to healthy food in your home. Maybe you have an overscheduled life or highly demanding job. Maybe your cultural background makes you more prone to gaining weight.

No matter what, we're all different.

With that said, I hope you see the power in the **10 Proven Secrets**, because if you practice them as I have shared them here, they will make a difference in your life and your weight.

Don't fall for the hype that says that you can buy this weight loss pill or this exercise machine or this workout DVD and you'll be skinny by Monday. It just isn't true.

By focusing on the psychology of weight loss and how to harness your emotions for the best power when it comes to losing weight, you'll be able to have a long-term effect on your body that many people never realize.

Take a look at some other behavioral strategies that you can use to help you lose weight and keep it off.

Communication: Believe it or not, asking for support from your family and friends can be one of the best things you do for losing weight. Sometimes people try to do it on their own without telling everyone, and that may work if you have a very unsupportive group of family and friends. If you don't have supportive family and friends, get some! Find people who can encourage you and support you through the process even if it means that you join some kind of weight loss or health support group.

Schedule your day: One of the biggest problems with losing weight for many people is overscheduled lives. Set your alarm early so that you can get up and exercise. Simply scheduling your day, and prioritizing what's important can make a huge difference in your weight loss progress.

Buy healthy snacks: It might sound very simplistic, but you need to have healthy snacks around so your food choices when you are hungry will support your goals and intentions. Get nuts, carrots or organic grapes, etc. Make sure that you have plenty of protein with your snacks and meals so you'll stay full longer and stoke your metabolism.

Create a vision board: You might want to have a vision board with some old pictures of you when you were at your target weight. Even if you never were at your target weight, you can have pictures of other people. Be realistic here. Don't put supermodels on your vision board as you're likely to never attain that Photoshop physique. However, you might want to post pictures of healthy foods, people doing exercise or whatever it is that you'd like to do once you get down to your healthy weight.

Stay in the moment: This refers back to what we talked about earlier which is not to eat in front of the TV, while you're working on the computer, or while you're driving down the road. Don't multitask when you're eating. Instead, savor each bite and feel what fullness actually feels like.

Here's another important point to remember that derails a lot of people in the weight loss journey. Make sure that you're not focusing on your past diets or weight loss failure as a negative thing.

We have to learn to be able take what we can from our mistakes and use it to make ourselves stronger. Beating yourself up over something is not going to help you avoid repeating history. No one is perfect, and today is a new day.

Today you have **10 Proven Secrets** that have the power to help you achieve a healthy weight permanently, IF you practice these **10 Proven Secrets** every day, and repeat them as outlined in this book.

When it comes to losing weight, the main determining factor of your weight loss has more to do with how you think, your attitude, your mindset and finally the decisions that you make than it does about whether or not you get on that recumbent bike this afternoon after work. You can get on that recumbent bike and go 5 miles a day, but the moment that you hit an emotional issue that you can't solve without eating a piece of chocolate cake, you're starting the beginning cycle all over again anyway.

Here's the thing: you would think that with that such a fast-paced, technologically advanced society that we would not have any weight problems anymore. We've never been more educated than we are right now. We've never had more advanced medical care or more food options or more weight loss programs than we do right now. And yet, we've never been fatter as a society.

We have all the resources we could ever want or need, yet more people make excuses instead of working to get healthy. Why is this?

I would venture to say that it's due in part to the fact that we look for the "quick fix". Rarely do people go through the psychological process to change how they think about food, hunger, and health before they attempt to lose weight.

We do a lot of things *mindlessly* throughout the day. Being mindful, intentional, and truly listening to our body are all steps that will shift us to success in this journey.

Weight loss and attaining a healthy weight happens above your shoulders first.

Yes, losing weight will require some effort on your part in the way of exercise. However, if you're doing exercise or movement that you absolutely love to do and look forward to, it's no longer a chore.

I personally love my rebounder/mini trampoline. I grab my iPod with my favorite tunes and jump to my heart's delight – literally. It's low impact, fun, and very good for you.

Why do we think that weight loss has to be a punishment? That is one of the biggest emotional issues that I see in people. They believe that they have to punish themselves by starving and doing exercises that they hate.

It's really quite the opposite – this can truly be one of the most *amazing* journeys you've ever embarked upon!

22 ADDITIONAL TIPS THAT SUPPORT EASY WEIGHT LOSS

As with anything, it makes sense to have as many tools in your arsenal as possible. While I'm not going to give you specific foods to eat or not eat or even specific exercises that you should do, I do want to give you some more tips that will help you in your weight loss journey. These tips may go without saying, but when you put them into practice along with the **10 Proven Secrets** outlined here, you will see success even faster.

The end result that I want to see for you is not only weight loss, but long-lasting health and the power to keep the weight off without dietary restrictions or stress. After all, who wants to spend the rest of their life counting calories and sweating for hours each day? Not me – and probably not you.

We pretty much all know that 1 pound of fat is equal to 3500 calories. Simply knocking 500 calories a day off through movement and dietary changes will allow you to lose at least a pound a week. So, you can see that making substantial changes to the way that you think and approach food, you to lose weight at a rapid clip.

Add to that the fact that you can incorporate exercises into your daily routine that you actually enjoy, and you could become a fat burning furnace in no time. Let's take a look at some of the things you could do to help quicken the process of losing weight.

Eat breakfast: It's very important that you get into the habit of eating breakfast every single day. Almost anyone who is having success at losing weight and keeping it off say that they eat breakfast. When I say breakfast, I don't mean for you to grab a glazed doughnut and a cup of coffee on your way to work. Again, you have to follow the **10 Proven Secrets** outlined here - sit down, savor your food slowly, pay special attention to when you're satisfied, etc.

Studies actually show that people who eat breakfast have a lower BMI than people who skip breakfast. In addition, eating breakfast will allow you to perform better at work or school. Obviously, loading yourself up with empty calories and sugar is going to cause a crash later and make you tired and shaky.

As you tune in to your body and really listen, many of these things change naturally *because you want them to.*

Some healthy options for breakfast include whole-grain cereals, eggs and anything else that will give you the protein boost that you need for your metabolism at the start of the day.

It's worth mentioning that you should also eat something before you exercise first thing in the morning. This is an important part of making sure that your body has the fuel that it needs for the movement that it requires. I personally love a small amount of fat-free Greek yoghurt with a small amount of fruit.

Liquid calories: Enjoy the foods and beverages that you love. I stand by this statement. With that said, you want to make sure that you are also getting plenty of water and not overdoing it with any specific beverage. If you're constantly drinking cola or sweet tea but not getting enough water, you are drinking in most of your calories not to mention dehydrating your body. Water is critical for detoxification, so make sure that you're getting more water than you are any other beverage. I don't drink any soda, not even diet. I consider them to be empty calories and not worth my time.

Produce: Choosing high-volume, filling fruits and vegetables that are low in calories will help you to shed the pounds more quickly. I personally eat organically, but if you don't, at least make sure you wash your foods before eating them to remove as much of the chemical and pesticide residue as possible.

Add a wide variety of vegetables and fruits into your diet so that you get plenty of vitamins and nutrients in your body. Believe me, when you start adding more vitamins, minerals and other nutrients to your body, it will quickly start to repair itself and help shed those extra pounds.

Stock your kitchen with fruits and vegetables. You don't have to spend a lot of money to get fruits and vegetables if you visit your local farmer's market or start growing some of your own. The more nutritious foods you eat, the less likely you are to crave unhealthy food. By getting your fruits and vegetables locally, you are getting more nutrients since your produce hasn't been sitting on a truck for days or weeks.

Why does this matter? The more that you can use your brain in weight loss, the better. How does produce factor into this? First, it gives you more nutrients that are critical for proper brain function and neurotransmitter production/balance. Secondly, part of using your brain means that you must use logic when eating. When you fill up on healthier options, you have room for your favorites too, but you won't eat as much of them.

Environment matters: I'm not going to tell you to keep snacks and other fun foods out of your kitchen. Instead, I want to encourage you to focus on the environment that you set for yourself when you're about to eat. Many of us keep our kitchen tables piled with the mail and other clutter, but we don't sit there to eat our breakfast, lunch and dinner. Because of this, you may have a hard time sitting down for a meal as outlined here.

Take control of your environment by creating a place where you *enjoy* eating. Buy a nice new tablecloth, set your table, put a candle in the middle. You might even want to get fresh flowers once per week so you can enjoy the eating experience even more. When you set up an environment that you enjoy and that makes you feel like you are in a fine dining restaurant, you will actually begin to look forward to your meals whether you are alone or with family.

By setting up an environment that you enjoy, you'll be less tempted to sit down in front of the TV with plates of food you can eat mindlessly. Turn on some soft music if you want, but do get in the habit of sitting at the table, eating slowly and enjoying every bite.

Get a pedometer: A pedometer is a very inexpensive way to monitor the number of steps that you're taking each day. Set a goal of 5,000 and then 10,000 steps per day. By using a pedometer, you'll get a better idea of how much you are actually moving during the day so that you can continue to increase that as you desire.

You can use your pedometer during any kind of activity, even walking! You can purchase a pedometer for less than five dollars in many big box retail stores.

Time your meals: You may not understand what slow eating really means. Buy an inexpensive kitchen timer or use the one on your microwave oven to make sure that you spend at least 20 to 30 minutes eating your meal. This will allow you to savor each bite and not hurry through. As you get to the 20-minute mark, your body's full notification will come from its hormones and will keep you from wanting to overeat. Strive to take the full 20 to 30 minutes of time instead of rushing through you meals. Believe it or not, many people can finish a meal in 5 or 10 minutes sitting in front of the TV which causes them to crave other foods later simply because they did not get that "full" signal from slower eating.

Get plenty of sleep: Did you know that an extra hour of sleep per night can help a person drop 14 pounds in a year? A University of Michigan researcher looked at the numbers for a 2500-calorie per day intake. When you get enough sleep, you're well rested and not as tempted to eat out of emotions during the day. Sleep gives you more energy to work out, and helps your body maintain its hormonal balance, thus making weight loss easier and weight gain less likely.

Buy your dream outfit: Buy a dress, a pair of pants or some other outfit that is the target goal for you. Hang it up where you can see it every day as you get ready for work. This will allow you to stay focused on the goal of a healthy weight.

Smaller plates: Some people like to use smaller plates in order to eat foods they love without eating such huge portions. There is also no question that restaurants give us portions that are way too large, so it also makes sense to ask for a to-go box as soon as you get your meal. Simply split it in half, or ask for a half portion when you order. At home, you can use salad plates in place of dinner plates to cut your portion sizes immediately.

With this program, if you're still hungry at the end of your relaxed 20-30 minute meal, you can always order or add additional food. But the odds are – you won't be hungry.

Try yoga: According to the American Dietetic Association, women who do yoga actually tend to weigh less than others. This is because yoga allows you to slow down and learn how to use mindfulness. A mindful approach to eating leads to higher self-awareness and helps us resist emotional eating patterns.

Put your fork down between bites: Many people who have been successful at losing weight and keeping it off report that when they put the fork down between bites, it allows them to savor the food and take their time eating it. It's just another way to support mindful eating.

Don't skip meals: It might be very tempting to skip meals when trying to accelerate weight loss, but it's actually unhealthy and often does the opposite of what you're seeking. Skipping meals can make your body go into starvation mode, which makes it even harder to burn calories. You don't have to eat huge meals 5 or 6 times per day – just remember that when your body signals hunger it is read to metabolize what you eat. Eat only until you are satisfied and then move on with your day.

Be careful with grocery shopping: <u>Never</u> go grocery shopping when you're hungry. This will cause you to buy all kinds of things you may not normally purchase. Take a shopping list and set a time limit for your shopping trip. Of course, if you see something that you really love to eat, don't be afraid to get it. As long as you follow the rules outlined here, it will be okay. Focus on creating a shopping cart full of colors and the nutrients that your body needs for fuel. Choose fresher, whole food and less boxed and processed stuff.

Thirst: A lot of people confuse thirst with hunger. By drinking that important glass of pure water when you feel hungry, you be able to see if you really craving liquid or food. Dehydration can actually make you feel hungry rather than thirsty. By the time you are thirsty, you are already at least slightly dehydrated. Drink pure water throughout the day, before meals to make sure that your body is getting plenty of water.

Take a walk before lunch or dinner: When you exercise before you eat, you are less likely to choose unhealthy options. No one wants to throw away the benefits of exercise that they've done, so you're more likely to reinforce good choices. Additionally, walking revs your metabolism and calms you down. All of these support weight loss.

Separate your snacks: This is another great rule to follow. Don't eat any snack food straight out-of-the-box, bag or carton that they came in. You will be much less likely to overeat if you separate your snacks into fist size servings. Put them in Ziploc bags so that you can have easy access to them when you're hungry.

Eat proteins before a workout: You might want to try a protein-fused smoothie or Greek yogurt with frozen berries before you do your workout. This will help you have more stamina and burn fat rather than muscle mass.

Avoid eating late at night: You've probably heard many researchers and doctors say that you should not eat past 6 PM or 7 PM or 8 PM at night. Again, if you're hungry, just follow the secrets outlined as a way to taper your eating. However, many times we eat at night simply out of boredom or emotional issues. Instead, make sure that you are thinking through what you're doing before you eat late at night.

Here's why. When you go to bed your digestive system needs to shut down for a while to give it time to detoxify your body and rest. When you eat, you're giving your digestive system *extra* things to do in the middle of the night. To avoid these digestive disturbances and extra weight gain, try not to eat late at night or at least pick some healthy options that are easy to digest such as a banana or grapes.

Take a 30 second break: In the middle of your meal, about 10 or 15 minutes in, take a 30 second break to evaluate how hungry you really are before you get back to eating your food. Often, once you check in with yourself you'll see that you are potentially already satisfied.

Fit exercise into your day: If you are going to watch TV, use the commercial breaks as opportunities to exercise. Here are some ideas: keep some resistance bands nearby (or even at work so you can do some weight training while you are sitting at your desk). Take the stairs as often as you can. Walk or ride your bike to work if it's a short distance. Do some squats during breaks. Make friends that are physically active so that you can get involved in physical activities. Offer to walk the dogs at the local animal shelter. Whatever you do, make it something that you enjoy and can fit into your day. All of these little exercise sessions can make a big difference in your overall calorie burn and health.

Don't compare yourself to other people: As we talked about before, everyone is unique. Everyone has different challenges, environmental triggers and emotional triggers. Your body is not going to always respond the same as your friend or family member. Focus on yourself and improving what you can about your own life and body. Set your goals, and stay focused on what *you* want to achieve.

Take a 30-day break from sugar: The **10 Proven Secrets To Permanent Weight Loss** will work without this step, and it will work *more quickly* with it. If you commit to going without sugar for 30 days, it will change your life. I personally found that I had more energy, control, and even insight at the end of my "sugar fast" as I called it. I highly recommend this step, if only as a step of empowerment. Sugar is addictive, and our body does not need it. (NOTE: I did eat organic fruit during this time. I allowed any *whole food* that naturally contained sugar.)

CONCLUSION – PRACTICE THE 10 PROVEN SECRETS EVERY DAY

As you can see, this book is probably different from any other weight-loss book you've read. Instead of outlining what foods you need to eat, I'm telling you to eat whatever you love. I'm telling you there's no forbidden food! Isn't that amazing?

I'm also not telling you how much weight to lift in the gym or the kind of exercises to do.

Do what you enjoy. Move your body. It knows what to do if you give it what it needs – if you listen.

Find things that you LOVE. This is about loving your life – NOT drudging through your day eating rice cakes because some weight loss guru told you it had to be that way. It's about using your brain, retraining how you think, and removing those emotional eating cues that get you off course.

Our ancestors didn't have to eat a specific diet or make sure that they walked a certain number of miles per day. They just ate when they were hungry and walked and moved around throughout most of their day. We can learn a lot from them. They knew what physical hunger felt like, and they followed what their bodies told them to do. They were not obsessed with food like we are in our media-focused culture today.

Put the 10 Proven Secrets into practice in your life starting right now.

Your weight will naturally go to the number on the scale that it's supposed to be over time. You won't have to worry about it or obsess over it anymore. You won't have to count calories or points. You won't have to read a bunch of weight loss books or join programs and talk to weight loss counselors.

Everything that you need to lose weight is not at the gym down the street. Instead, it is within you. Choose to follow the **10 Proven Secrets** as outlined here, and you too can realize a life that is more free, healthy and happy!

Take control and use mindfulness and intention as an asset in your weight loss journey, you will see results faster – and results that will last for a lifetime.

Fads and crash diets will be a thing of the past for you as you focus on *loving the food you eat* and living a more energized life!

THANK YOU – BOOK BONUS!

I hope you have enjoyed **10 Proven Secrets To Permanent Weight Loss!**

Please stop by my website: http://ElleGarner.com/Bonus to download your free copy of the **10 Proven Secrets Steps PDF**, formatted and ready for you to print! **You will need this password to unlock the bonus: **10secrets** (it is case sensitive, so please type the password in exactly as shown).

** If you liked this book (or even if you didn't), please consider putting a review on Amazon, and connect with me there!

You can put a copy on your refrigerator, keep a printed copy on your nightstand, in your briefcase or handbag, and print as many copies as you need to remind you to follow the **10 Proven Secrets** all day, *every* day.

I sincerely hope you will take these **10 Proven Secrets** seriously. Just Try It! Do it for 30-days, and then I believe it will become your life pattern as you begin to see the amazing, liberating **Power** in these **Secrets**.

Remember -- **You Can Do This!** I'm living proof.

Best wishes for a healthier, slimmer, happier YOU.

~Elle

Other Books by Elle Garner: <u>*Drink Pure Water: Pure Water and Hydration are Critical for Performance, Weight Loss, and Health. Learn Why – and Where to Find it, Make it, and Get it.*</u>